Siddharth Verma

Iontophoretic Drug Delivery System

Iontophoresis

LAP LAMBERT Academic Publishing

Impressum/Imprint (nur für Deutschland/only for Germany)
Bibliografische Information der Deutschen Nationalbibliothek: Die Deutsche Nationalbibliothek verzeichnet diese Publikation in der Deutschen Nationalbibliografie; detaillierte bibliografische Daten sind im Internet über http://dnb.d-nb.de abrufbar.
Alle in diesem Buch genannten Marken und Produktnamen unterliegen warenzeichen-, marken- oder patentrechtlichem Schutz bzw. sind Warenzeichen oder eingetragene Warenzeichen der jeweiligen Inhaber. Die Wiedergabe von Marken, Produktnamen, Gebrauchsnamen, Handelsnamen, Warenbezeichnungen u.s.w. in diesem Werk berechtigt auch ohne besondere Kennzeichnung nicht zu der Annahme, dass solche Namen im Sinne der Warenzeichen- und Markenschutzgesetzgebung als frei zu betrachten wären und daher von jedermann benutzt werden dürften.

Coverbild: www.ingimage.com

Verlag: LAP LAMBERT Academic Publishing GmbH & Co. KG
Heinrich-Böcking-Str. 6-8, 66121 Saarbrücken, Deutschland
Telefon +49 681 3720-310, Telefax +49 681 3720-3109
Email: info@lap-publishing.com

Herstellung in Deutschland (siehe letzte Seite)
ISBN: 978-3-8484-8908-4

Imprint (only for USA, GB)
Bibliographic information published by the Deutsche Nationalbibliothek: The Deutsche Nationalbibliothek lists this publication in the Deutsche Nationalbibliografie; detailed bibliographic data are available in the Internet at http://dnb.d-nb.de.
Any brand names and product names mentioned in this book are subject to trademark, brand or patent protection and are trademarks or registered trademarks of their respective holders. The use of brand names, product names, common names, trade names, product descriptions etc. even without a particular marking in this works is in no way to be construed to mean that such names may be regarded as unrestricted in respect of trademark and brand protection legislation and could thus be used by anyone.

Cover image: www.ingimage.com

Publisher: LAP LAMBERT Academic Publishing GmbH & Co. KG
Heinrich-Böcking-Str. 6-8, 66121 Saarbrücken, Germany
Phone +49 681 3720-310, Fax +49 681 3720-3109
Email: info@lap-publishing.com

Printed in the U.S.A.
Printed in the U.K. by (see last page)
ISBN: 978-3-8484-8908-4

TABLE OF CONTENTS

[1] INTRODUCTION

Iontophoretic drug delivery is an accepted method of drug therapy which is gaining wide popularity especially in the area of pain relief. This technique provides a means for regulated non-invasive systemic administration of minute amounts of drug transdermally which is especially useful in patients who require long-term medication as in chronic pain, diabetics, hypertensives, rheumatoids etc. It negates the need for needle sticks, the pain and anxiety involved and minimises the trauma and risks of infection associated with it. This mode of drug delivery is simple, versatile, effective, reliable and can be tailored for individual needs[1].

There has been a growing awareness in recent years of potential therapeutic importance of achieving true controlled drug delivery where the rate of drug output may be modulated in a precisely controlled manner. Transdermal drug delivery has usefulness in achieving the controlled delivery of pharmaceuticals, which are relatively small in molecular size and rather lipophilic in nature, however, these systems are rather limited in their capability of achieving the transdermal systemic delivery of peptides, proteins and drugs which is often charged and highly hydrophilic in nature. In order to deliver an ionic drug, peptide/protein molecule through transdermal delivery to attain a systemic effect, chemical and/or physical methods are required to enhance the rate of penetration of therapeutic agent through the main diffusion barrier. The iontophoretic technique is highly desirable to improve the transdermal delivery of peptide and proteins using a lower current intensity with a short time period. The idea of applying electric current to increase the penetration of electrically charged drugs into surface tissues was probably organized by *Veratti* in 1947. *Leduc* did the first well-documented experiments at the beginning of the 20th century. Leduc demonstrated the introduction of strychnine and cyanide ions into the rabbits when the correct polarities were applied.

Inchley also carried out similar experiments in 1921. The application of iontophoresis to the treatment of hyperhydrosis could be reduced by ion transfer of certain applied solutions by electro-phoretic technique. Today, the treatment of hyperhydrosis is the most successful and popular applications of iontophoresis in dermatological medication. The transdermal delivery of many ionized drugs at therapeutic levels is precluded by their slow rate of diffusion under a concentration gradient alone are now application with the help of iontophoretic technique and devices.

Iontophoresis can be defined as the process in which the flux or rate of absorption of ionic solutes into or through skin is enhanced by applying a voltage drop/electric field across the skin. Transdermal iontophoretic technique is capable of administering drugs in a pulsatile pattern by alternately applying and terminating the current input at programmed rate. In addition, delivery rate can be controlled by the intensity of applied electric current or Electro-chemical potential gradient. It can also be define as a means of enhancing the flux of ionic drugs across skin by the application of an electrochemical potential gradient.

Trans-dermal administration of drug is assuming an important place in modern drug therapy. It is used for non-ionized drugs required in a small dosage. Trans-dermal administration can be passive or facilitated. In passive administration, the non-ionized drug traverses the skin through the stratum corneum. The skin, being a semi-permeable membrane, allows only a small amount of any drug molecule to passively penetrate the skin. Ionized drugs do not easily penetrate this barrier and are not suitable for routine trans-dermal delivery unless an external source of energy is provided to drive the drug across the skin. Facilitated diffusion can utilize either ultrasound (phonophoresis) or electrical (iontophoresis) energy. In iontophoresis, this external source of energy is in the form of an applied direct electrical current[2].

1.1 Iontophoresis

The Greek ion or **Iontos** refers to an atom having negative or a positive charge as a results of the loss or gain one or more electrons. **Phoresis** refers to being carried. A direct electric current provides the electromotive force to move the ionized particle of the drug past the barrier of the skin and into the deeper layer tissue. The route of entry is through the pores,the sweat glands, and the hair follicles. In addition, the overall resistance of the skin will decrease somewhat under the influence of electricity, allowing further passive passage of the drug into the dermal layer.

Different investigators have given different definitions because one simple definition cannot explain all the mechanisms involved. But for the sake of simplicity,

"Iontophoresis is a process of transportation of ionic molecules into the tissues by passage of electric current through the electrolyte solution containing the ionic molecules using a suitable electrode polarity." This means it would involve an electromotive force. In the body, ions with a positive charge (+) are driven into the skin at the anode and those with negative charge (-) at the cathode.

Iontophoresis is sometimes confused with electrophoresis and electro-osmosis, the former involving movement of the colloid (dispersed phase) and the latter involving the liquid (dispersion medium), which are quite different. Iontophoresis may however cause an increased transport of method of penetration of non electrolytes through tissues.

Iontophoresis is defined as the topical introduction of ionized drugs into the skin using direct current. However, Iontophoresis treatment with simple tap water alone is successful in a vast majority of people who suffer from hyperhidrosis of the hands and feet[3].

[2] IONTOPHORETIC ELECTROCHEMISTRY

An iontophoretic device comprises a power source and two electrode compartments. The drug formulation (D^+A^-) containing the ionized molecule (D^+) is placed in the electrode compartment bearing the same charge; for example, a positively charged drug such as lidocaine would be placed in the anodal compartment. The indifferent electrode compartment is placed at a distal site on the skin. Although there are many different types of electrode, the most well-suited to iontophoresis is the Ag/AgCl couple [4–6]. First, it avoids the sharp decreases in pH that are seen with, for example, Pt-metal electrodes: Ag/AgCl electrodes have the considerable advantage that their electrochemistry occurs at voltages lower than those necessary for the electrolysis of water, which is undesirable for two reasons: first, the protons created at the anode compete to carry charge and because of their small size and high mobility, they may significantly reduce drug delivery efficiency, and second, the low pH produced in the anodal compartment can lead to acid-induced skin burns and it may have an adverse effect on drug stability. Once the current is applied, the electric field imposes a directionality on the movements of the ions present: positive charges in the anodal compartment move towards the cathode whereas anions move in the opposite direction. The electrochemistry occurring at the Ag anode necessitates the presence of Cl^- ions in the anodal compartment: this requirement usually leads to a decrease in drug delivery efficiency since the NaCl commonly used to provide Cl^- also introduces significant concentrations of highly mobile Na^+ ions which compete very effectively with the drug to carry current. As the Cl^- ions arrive at the electrode solution interface, they react with the metallic silver to form silver chloride, which on account of its low solubility product, is deposited at the electrode surface, simultaneously releasing an electron. In order to maintain electroneutrality in the anodal compartment, either a cation must move out of the compartment and into the skin or an anion must leave the skin and move into the anodal chamber. In the cathodal compartment, the AgCl is reduced by the arrival of electrons from the power supply and yields metallic silver together with a Cl^- ion, which passes into the solution. Again, for electroneutrality, this must be compensated for by the arrival of a cation from within the skin into the cathodal chamber or by the loss of an anion. Since the electrical circuit is completed by the endogenous inorganic ions that are present in the skin, primarily Na^+ and Cl^-, these latter species can impact on the efficiency of drug transport[4].

[3] MECHANISM OF IONTOPHORESIS

In the iontophoresis process, the current, beginning at the device, is transferred from the electrode through the ionized drug solution as ionic flow.

The drug ions are moved to the skin where the repulsion continues moving the drug through the trans-appendageal structures and stratum corneum interstices via the aqueous pores.

The larger the electrode surface, the greater the current the device must supply to provide a current density for moving the drug.

Iontophoresis enhances transdermal drug delivery by three mechanisms:

(a)   Ion-electric field interaction provides an additional force that drives ions through the skin,

(b)   The flow of electric current increases the permeability of the skin, and

(c)   Electro-osmosis produces bulk motion of solvent that carries ions or neutral species with the solvent stream.

Electro-osmotic flow occurs in a variety of membranes and is in the same direction as the flow of counter-ions.

It may assist or hinder drug transport. Since human skin is negatively charged above pH 4, counter ions are positive ions and electro-osmotic flow occurs from anode to cathode. Thus, anodic delivery is assisted by electro-osmosis but cathodic delivery is retarded.

Because of the electro-osmotic flow, transdermal delivery of a large anion (negatively charged protein) from the anode compartment is more effective than that from the cathode compartment.

In order to deliver a positively charged drug across the skin, a solution of, for example, a cationic drug is placed at the positive electrode where it is repelled and then attracted towards a negative electrode place elsewhere on the body.

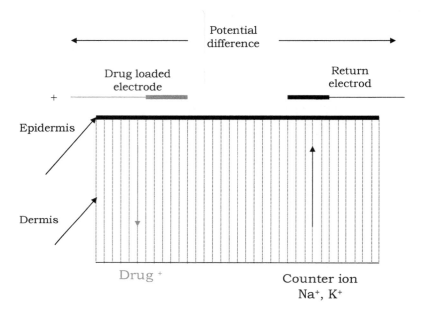

Iontophoretic delivery of positively charged ion through skin

Delivery of positively charged compounds is generally easier than negatively charged compounds as the skin itself possesses a net negative charge[5].

[4] PRINCIPLES OF IONTOPHORETIC TREATMENT

Iontophoresis increases the penetration of electrically charged drugs into surface tissues by the application of an electric current. Electrical energy assists the movement of ions across the stratum corneum according to the basic electrical principle of "like charges repel each other and opposite charges attract".

Iontophoresis is a no-invasive drug system. By applying a low-level electrical current to a similarly charged drug solution. Iontophoresis repels the drug ions through the skin to the underlying tissue. In contrast to passive transdermal patch drug delivery, iontophoresis is active (electrical driven) method that allows the delivery of water-soluble ionic drugs that are not effectively absorbed through the skin. One of the patch's gel reservoirs is prefilled with a drug. Drugs with a positive charge are placed in positive reservoir. When the patch is applied to the skin, the preprogrammed microprocessor and battery indicate an electric current between the electrodes. An ion exchange between the electrode and the drugs forces the drug into the skin. An opposite reaction at the return electrode completes the electrical circuit. The range of drugs that can be delivered transdermally is greatly expanded. Iontophoresis has the capability of delivering up to 50mg (under 500 mol w) per day of small drug such as: lidocain, a topical anesthetic- and larger drugs such as: peptides with a 3500 mol wt.

The drug is applied under an electrode of the same charge as the drug, and a return electrode opposite in charge to the drug is placed at a neutral site on the body surface. The operator then selects a current below the level of the patient's pain threshold and allows it to flow for an appropriate length of time. The electrical current significantly increases the penetration of the drug into surface tissues by repulsion of like charges and attraction of opposite charges. The two classically considered prerequisites for iontophoretic treatment are that the drug must be charged (or modified to carry a charge) and that the disease process must be at or near a body surface[6].

[5] IONTOPHORESIS OF NON-PEPTIDIC THERAPEUTIC AGENTS

5.1. Pain management

Iontophoresis has obvious applications in pain management—appropriate modulation of the current profile means that iontophoresis can provide relief in response to acute pain episodes, e.g. post-operative pain and also alleviate chronic pain, e.g. in cancer patients. The current controlled input kinetics allows the non invasive administration of bolus doses as with conventional, but more invasive patient-controlled anesthesia devices; in addition, maintenance doses can be achieved using a continuous current profile. Furthermore, as well as providing systemic pain relief, iontophoresis can also be used for local pain relief or local anesthesia prior to minor surgical procedures[7].

5.1.1. Opioids

Opioid analgesics have molecular weights in the range of 300–500 Da and under physiological conditions, the molecules are usually positively charged. In addition, they are capable of eliciting a pharmacological effect at relatively low systemic concentrations, typically in the mg ml^{-1} range. These physicochemical and pharmacological properties make these molecules candidates for iontophoretic delivery. Ashburn and coworkers used the Iomed PhoresorR (a "fill on site" device that uses a Ag / AgCl anode) to study the iontophoretic delivery of morphine (in the form of its hydrochloride) in vivo in humans. A group of post-surgical patients was initially placed on IV meperidine; they were then divided into two subgroups, one of which received iontophoretic morphine for a period of 6 h at the current required to deliver an equianalgesic dose to the meperidine infusion (morphine input rate 1.3 mg mA^{-1} h^{-1}), while the control group received buffer (lactated ringer solution). The patient controlled anesthesia (PCA) option remained available to both sets of patients and the results demonstrated that the iontophoretic group made fewer requests for PCA than the control group. The authors also measured the blood concentrations of unbound morphine in the iontophoretic sample group and showed that minimally effective concentrations of morphine (f20 mg ml^{-1}) were attained within 30 min of commencing iontophoresis and levels capable of providing consistent pain relief (f40 mg ml^{-1}) were achieved during current application. Patients in the iontophoretic group displayed a red wheal and flare under and around the anodal compartment: this was attributed to local histamine release provoked by the opioid. Stephens et al. investigated the iontophoretic delivery of morphine citrate in the presence and absence of sodium citrate buffer as part of an in vivo human study. In contrast to the investigation by Ashburn et al., they used a carbon anode, proposing that the presence of the sodium citrate buffer would serve to "mop up" the protons created at the anode. A 2 mA pulsed DC current (2.5 kHz) was applied for 58 min (after an initial 2 min ramping-up period) to a formulation containing 9.4 mg ml^{-1} morphine (f33 mM). Their results indeed showed a smaller pH decrease when the formulation in the anodal compartment contained sodium citrate (a drop from pH 6 to 5.3 in the presence of buffer as compared to 6 to 4.3 in its absence). Slightly higher blood levels of morphine were found in the presence of the sodium citrate buffer. Although it is certainly true that the citrate would eliminate competition from the protons generated at the anode, the sodium counter-ions would also compete with the bulkier morphine cations and would carry a significant fraction of the charge. Since the donor compartment pH was higher in the presence of the citrate buffer (5.0–6.2 vs. 4.0–5.4), the authors suggested that the increased delivery was perhaps due to the presence of a second "electrokinetic phenomenon", which they referred to as electrophoresis, and,which is most likely electroosmosis. Subsequent studies by other groups have shown that the isoelectric point of skin is at pH 4–4.5 ; therefore, it is indeed possible that iontophoresis of morphine, in the absence of buffer, results in a neutralization of skin charge and inhibition of electroosmosis. Although the iontophoretic delivery of morphine was shown to be feasible by these studies, the plasma levels attained were at the lower limits of those generally regarded as necessary for consistent pain relief. Research into the iontophoretic delivery of morphine has been superseded by the advent of more potent opioids with lower minimum therapeutic plasma concentrations. Like morphine, fentanyl, a 4-anilidopiperidine, is also positively charged at physiological pH; however, it has a much greater affinity for the mu-opioid receptor and is a significantly more potent analgesic than morphine—estimates attribute fentanyl activities ranging from 100 to 500 times that of morphine. Consequently, the therapeutic levels necessary to produce analgesia are much lower (1–3 mg ml^{-1}). Furthermore, it is subject to a considerable hepatic first-pass effect and has a short half-life. These properties coupled with a narrow therapeutic index make it an attractive candidate for iontophoresis and there have been several reports in the literature describing its electrically assisted delivery both in vitro and in vivo. *Thysman et al.* conducted a detailed investigation of the influence of experimental parameters, including the current profile, current intensity, drug concentration and formulation pH on the iontophoresis of fentanyl and sufentanil across rat skin in vitro using both direct and pulsed current profiles. Their results showed that iontophoretic transport was proportional to the applied current, with 3-fold increases in current intensity ($0.17–0.5$ mA cm^{-2}) producing 2–3-fold increases in drug flux. However, a 10-fold increase in drug concentration only resulted in a 2-fold increase in drug flux. This non-linear response may be due to these lipophilic cations binding to the skin to form a reservoir within the cutaneous membrane. This would also explain why drug permeation across the skin continues after termination of the current. The authors also found higher delivery at lower pH (3.5 vs. 7.0), which was somewhat surprising given that these drugs are >95% ionized at pH 7.0 and iontophoretic transport at this pH should also benefit from an electroosmotic contribution. In a subsequent in vivo study in rats, the authors demonstrated that appreciable plasma concen- trations of both fentanyl and sufentanil could be achieved by iontophoresis (Cmax of 29.3F14 and 29.1F9.9 mg ml^{-1} for fentanyl and sufentanil, respectively). Ashburn et al. showed that therapeutically relevant plasma concentrations of fentanyl (Cmaxf1.6F0.2 ng ml^{-1}) could be achieved when the citrate salt was iontophoresed at a current of 2 mA min for 2 h in a group of five volunteers. Interestingly, unlike morphine, the iontophoretic delivery of fentanyl did not elicit a histamine response in the skin. More recently, Alza Corporation has developed its E-TRANSR electro-transport technology to provide a delivery platform for the iontophoretic administration of fentanyl as an alternative to more invasive methods of PCA. *Gupta et al.* have extensively investigated fentanyl pharmacokinetics following iontophoretic delivery in man as a function of the applied current and the input profile. They showed that when subjects received fentanyl continuously over a 24-h period from the E-TRANSR system (containing 10 mg of fentanyl imbibed in a gel; area = 5 cm^2) at 50, 100 and 200 AA, the maximum plasma concentrations increased in direct proportion to the applied current. The measured AUCs also increased with increasing current although they did not exhibit the same proportionality. In a second study, the subjects received a 20 min iontophoretic application using the E-TRANSR system (containing 5 mg of fentanyl imbibed in a gel; area = 2 cm^2) at the beginning of each hour over a 24-h period, and the pharmacokinetic parameters measured using 150, 200 and 250 AA were compared to an i.v. fusion (50 Ag) administered at the same time points and for an identical duration. The impressive results showed that iontophoretic delivery was more than able to match the IV input kinetics. Based on the amount of fentanyl delivered in the 20-min period during 24–25th h, it can be shown that fentanyl had a highly respectable transport number of f0.09, implying that it was responsible for approximately 10% of the total charge transferred during this period. *Padmanabhan et al.* conducted a detailed investigation of experimental parameters on the iontophoretic delivery of hydromorphone hydrochloride across excised porcine and human skin and in vivo in weanling pigs. The in vitro data demonstrated that although excised porcine skin was much more permeable than its human counterpart to the passive delivery of hydromorphone as evidenced by the input rates at steady state, the iontophoretic permeabilities were very similar. The authors also showed that although the delivery rate was linearly proportional to the applied current, the drug flux, in the absence of competing ions, was independent of drug concentration. The iontophoretic delivery efficiency, that is the amount of hydromorphone delivery per unit current per unit time was 1.1 and 1.2 mg h^{-1} mA^{-1} for porcine and human skin, respectively. This corresponds to a transport number of f0.11. In contrast to the in vitro studies, which were performed using conventional diffusion cells and aqueous media, the in vivo experiments were conducted using hydrogel electrode patches containing 3.2% hydromorphone hydrochloride (area = 25 cm^2). The current was applied for 12 h and the iontophoretic input rates were matched to an intravenous infusion. The invivo hydromorphone delivery rate, based on the plasma concentrations of the drug was higher than that observed in vitro (1.07F0.15 mg h^{-1} mA^{-1}) and that calculated from the residual amount of drug remaining in the patches; the authors tentatively proposed that this could be in part due to non-linear elimination kinetics of hydromorphone in the pig model. Buprenorphine is a partial agonist at the mu-receptor and a partial antagonist at the kappa-receptor. It is 20–50 times as potent as morphine and is indicated for the treatment of acute pain. It is administered parenterally owing to an extensive hepatic first pass effect, but even so, it has a short half-life and must be given three to four times per day. There have been reports describing the iontophoretic delivery of buprenorphine in vitro across skin from different animal species and across human skin. *Fang et al.* investigated buprenorphine iontophoresis across intact hairless mouse skin using current intensities of 0.3 and 0.5 mA cm^{-2}, which were each applied for 8 h. Their results showed that increasing the current had little effect on either the cumulative amount of buprenorphine delivered during iontophoresis or the flux across the membrane. Based on the cumulative amounts of drug recovered in the receiver compartment, it is possible to estimate a transport number of f0.001 for buprenorphine. *Bose et al.* also studied the iontophoresis of buprenorphine, using full-thickness porcine skin and human epidermal membrane. The cumulative amounts delivered after iontophoresing for 4 h at a current density of 0.5 mA cm^{-2} were approximately 2 and 30 Ag cm 2 for full thickness porcine skin and human epidermis, respectively. The human data suggest a transport number for buprenorphine of f0.0009, in close agreement with that found previously. After termination of the iontophoretic current, the authors also observed passive diffusion of buprenorphine across the skin as it was gradually released from (presumably) a reservoir in the skin (as was the case iontophoresis increased delivery with respect to passive diffusion across intact and impaired rodent skins, the flux across human skin showed only a very modest improvement over passive delivery[8].

5.1.2. NSAIDS

Although this is one of the most frequently administered classes of therapeutic agents, several drugs belonging to this category provoke harmful effects in the gastrointestinal tract after oral administration. The damage inflicted on the mucosa can result in ulceration and/or bleeding. Since the target compartment of these molecules is often an inflamed site, for example, muscle tissue, it is reasonable to assume that local administration would be a desirable option. Topical delivery would ensure that systemic concentrations would certainly be less than those observed following oral administration, hence reducing adverse secondary effects. In addition, the local concentrations at the target compartment may be higher leading to improved efficacy. These compounds are acidic and are usually negatively charged at physiological pH. Although effective passive transdermal delivery of the free base forms of these drugs has been achieved, it is logical that cathodal iontophoretic administration of the anionic forms of these drugs should be investigated as a means to improve both the rate and extent of drug delivery[8].

5.1.3. Local anesthetics

There have been several reports in the literature investigating the iontophoretic administration of lidocaine by iontophoresis. One of the earliest applications of topical lidocaine iontophoresis wasreported by *Gangarosa* for providing local anesthesia prior to tooth extraction or root canal surgery. Subsequently, other groups have investigated the ability of lidocaine iontophoresis to induce anesthesia in the skin and have compared its efficacy to topical application and/or subcutaneous infiltration prior to an intervention, e.g. insertion of a cannula. *Russo et al.* showed that although anesthesia induced by iontophoresis of 4% lidocaine solution for 6 min was, on average, of slightly shorter duration than that achieved by subcutaneous infiltration (14.5F9.5 vs. 22.2-7.3 min, respectively), it was nevertheless able to provide effective local anesthesia for a short period (f5 min) prior to an intervention. *Riviere et al.* used the isolated perfused porcine skin flap (ISPPF) model together with in vivo experiments in weanling pigs to quantify the effect of vasoactive compounds on lidocaine delivery. Their results demonstrated that vasodilators increased transdermal lidocaine flux and serum lidocaine concentrations by increasing venous efflux. Therefore, co-iontophoresis of a vasoconstrictor could be appropriate if depot or high local concentrations of lidocaine were required[9].

Irsfeld et al. compared the efficacity of anesthesia obtained in human volunteers after iontophoresis of a 5% lidocaine formulation containing 1:50000 adrenalinefor 10 min at a current density of 0.1–0.2 mA cm^{-2} with that observed following application of EMLA cream (a eutectic mixture of 2.5% lidocaine and 2.5% prilocaine). In this study, pain was induced in the volunteers by insertion of a 27-gauge cannula into a forearm vein. After this intervention, one group received lidocaine iontophoretically whereas EMLA was applied under occlusion in the second group. In the iontophoretic group, the pain was completely abolished in five out of six subjects after iontophoresis—much more rapidly than in the EMLA group. The fast onset that can be achieved by iontophoresis is one of the major advantages of iontophoresis over passive transdermal delivery. The presence of the vasoconstrictor ensured that effective lidocaine concentrations were maintained at the target site and meant that the duration of effect was comparable to that of EMLA. Furthermore, the depth of anesthesia within the skin was also found to be greater when using iontophoresis. Recently, two reports have been published describing lidocaine iontophoresis (2% lidocaine hydrochloride/ 1:100 000 epinephrine formulation for 10 min (maximum current of 20–40 mA min) in the pediatric population as a means to prevent pain associated with venipuncture. In the first study, iontophoresis was shown to be safe, effective and well-tolerated by the sample population of 6–17 year olds. The second study compared efficacy to EMLA for the insertion of IV cannulas in a similar group of subjects. Iontophoretic delivery produced equivalent dermal analgesia but with the added advantage of a more rapid onset[9].

5.1.4. Migraine

Jadoul et al. investigated the transdermal iontophoreticdelivery of alniditan, a 5-HT1D agonist developed to treat migraine headache. Alniditan has a molecular weight of f300 Da and is doubly positively charged at physiological pH (pKa 8.3 and 11.5), making it an interesting candidate for iontophoresis. The authors investigated the role of experimental parameters and found optimum delivery was achieved at pH 9.5 in 0.1 M borate buffer/0.007 M NaCl using 17 mM alniditan and this resulted in f600 Ag of the drug reaching the receiver compartment after 6 h of iontophoresis at 0.4 mA cm^{-2} (transport number f0.007). In a subsequent clinical study in human volunteers, alniditan (0.5 mg dispersed in a 10 cm^2 patch) was iontophoresed for 30 min after which the current was switched off before being restarted after a further 90 min and continued for another 30 min. The resulting plasma concentration showed two discrete peaks similar to the profile expected following repeated subcutaneous injection. The peak concentrations achieved were 4.49 and 5.37 mg ml^{-1}, respectively, and were bordering upon the therapeutic concentration range believed to be 5–20 mg ml^{-1}.

5.2 Neurodegenerative conditions:

5.2.1 Parkinson's and Alzheimer's disease

Hager et al. investigated the effect of using ethanol as a cosolvent to promote the iontophoretic delivery of a fused ring dopamine agonist with a molecular weight of 405 Da and a pKa of f7.5. Although the presence of ethanol produced a 5-fold increase in drug solubility, only a 2-fold increase in the iontophoretic delivery was observed—a cumulative amount of f 800 Ag cm^{-2} was delivered after 20 h of iontophoresis at 0.3 mA cm^{-2}, corresponding to a transport number of f0.009. However, a significantly greater amount (a 6–7-fold increase) was extracted from the skin. The authors suggested that the

CQA 206-291 precipitated out of solution as the ethanol diffused into the skin. Furthermore, it was also possible that although iontophoresis drove the ionized molecule into the skin, the CQA 206-291 exceeded its solubility limit within the membrane as it encountered Cl⁻ ions moving towards the anodal compartment. *Van der Geest et al.* conducted a detailed investigation into the iontophoretic delivery of R-apomorphine, which is a potent dopamine agonist. These preliminary experiments using human skin were designed to determine the dependence of the iontophoretic flux on the experimental parameters[10].

The authors demonstrated that the flux increased with increasing current density and the concentration of the drug in the donor compartment. The concentration dependence tended to approach a plateau as the solution concentration approached the solubility limit. The transport data showed that apomorphine had a transport number of f0.005, hence the more mobile Na⁺ and Cl⁻ ions, which were also present at higher concentrations than apomorphine, were the dominant charge carriers. The results also showed that a 2.3-fold higher flux was obtained on increasing the temperatures to 37 jC. In an interesting follow-up to the invitro study, the authors used their initial data to estimate the experimental parameters for an in vivo iontophoretic study in Parkinson's patients. The in vivo experiments were conducted using current intensities of 0.25 and 0.375 mA cm⁻², and with 20 cm² patches. Although measurable plasma apomorphine concentrations of 1.3F0.6 and 2.5F0.7 ng ml⁻¹, at 0.25 and 0.375 mA cm⁻², respectively, were achieved (corresponding to input fluxes of f18 and f30 Ag cm⁻² h⁻¹), these levels were sub-therapeutic. Ropinirole (MW 260.3 g mol⁻¹) is one of the newer dopamine agonists that has been introduced for the therapy of Parkinson's Disease. *Luzardo-Alvarez et al.* performed a mechanistic investigation into the iontophoretic delivery of ropinirole across weanling pig skin in vitro. The availability of ropinirole as a hydrochloride salt enabled the investigators to study the effect of current intensity and concentration on iontophoretic flux in the absence of competing ions in the donor compartment. Under these conditions it was shown that although the flux was essentially independent of drug concentration at a given current, significant and approximately proportionate increases in flux were observed with increasing current. *Kankkunen et al.* investigated the iontophoretic delivery of the reversible acetylcholinesterase inhibitor, tacrine, in human subjects. In order to maximize the transport efficiency of drug delivery, they used a novel two-compartment electrode system in which the drug reservoir was separated from the Ag/AgCl electrode and the NaCl necessary for electrode function, by a Nafion membrane. A current of 0.4 mA cm^{-2} was applied for 3 h to the ventral forearm using custom-made patches with an active surface area of 10 cm^2. The plasma tacrine concentrations measured after iontophoresis (14.9F2.6 mg ml^{-1}) compared favorably with those achieved with a commercially available device (21.3F5.9 mg ml^{-1}). Both values lie within the range of blood levels seen following oral administration of tacrine[10].

[6] IONTOPHORESIS OF PROTEINS AND PEPTIDES

6.1. Diabetes and insulin delivery

Monomeric human insulin consists of an A- (21 amino acids) and a B-chain (30 amino acids), and has a molecular weight of f6000 Da and is negatively charged. Electromigration of the peptide would obviously be facilitated by cathodal iontophoresis; however, the increasing importance of electroosmosis in the iontophoretic transport of high molecular weight species would perhaps also suggest a role for anodal delivery. Although there are some reports of successful anodal iontophoresis, *Langkjaer et al.* observed precipitate formation in the anodal chamber that was attributed to protein adsorption on the electrode surface followed by reduction of the disulfide bridges. In view of the huge potential market for a noninvasive insulin delivery system, it is not surprising that the iontophoretic delivery of insulin has long been viewed as the ''holy grail'' and there is a considerable body of work in this field. A number of fundamental in vitro studies have investigated the effect of iontophoretic parameters on insulin delivery and there have also been pharmacodynamic studies that have demonstrated the physiological effect of iontophoretically delivered insulin on blood glucose levels in different small animal models, usually mice, rats or rabbits. *Kari* used cathodal iontophoresis with currents ranging from 0.2 to 0.8 mA (patch area 6.2 cm2) applied for 2 h to deliver insulin to alloxan-diabetic rabbits whose stratum corneum had been removed prior to iontophoresis. Blood glucose levels clearly decreased as serum insulin concentrations increased. The results showed that although increasing the iontophoretic current from 0.2 to 0.4 mA produced a corresponding 3-fold increase in the serum insulin concentration, further increase to 0.8 mA had no effect. This was attributed to the generation of hydroxide ions at the electrode surface, which compete to carry the current in the cathodal compartment. Although these early studies prove that iontophoretic delivery of insulin is feasible in these animals (frequently after compromising the stratum corneum), the challenge is to extrapolate these results to humans where significantly greater quantities of the hormone are required for pharmacologic effect. A normal healthy individual produces 18–40 IU (where 1 IUf0.04 mg) of insulin per day, which corresponds to 0.2–0.5 IU kg^{-1} per day. Approximately half of this is secreted in the basal state and the rest is secreted in response to meals. Therefore, the basal secretion rate is f0.5–1.0 IU h^{-1}; an iontophoretic system would have to provide a drug input rate of 0.02–

0.04 mg h^{-1} to match the physiological rate of insulin secretion and for a 10 cm^2 patch, this equates to drug flux of 2–4 Ag cm^{-2} h^{-1}. Even this basal drug input exceeds the theoretical flux predicted for monomeric insulin based on the iontophoretic fluxes observed by *Green et al.* for low molecular weight anions. *Langkjaer et al.* observed significant enhancement of the iontophoretic flux of highly negatively charged monomeric insulin analogs across hairless mouse skin, even achieving the therapeutically relevant basal input rate described above, following an "ethanol-wipe" pretreatment. However, they added that the experiments needed to be repeated using either pig skin or human skin, before realistic conclusions could be drawn. From these calculations it is clear that simply achieving the basal insulin input rate is a challenge. Furthermore, in diabetic populations or in obese and insulin-resistant patients, the basal insulin requirement can be 2–4-fold higher (f2 IU kg^{-1} per day), posing further hurdles. In addition to the challenge of attaining the physiological levels of insulin required to elicit a pharmacologic response, its physicochemical properties are also not ideal for iontophoretic delivery. Insulin has a pI of f5.4; therefore, at a pH< 5.4, it has a net positive charge, whereas at pH>5.4 it is negatively charged. Bearing in mind that there is a pH gradient in the skin which goes from a weakly acidic f5 at the surface to a physiologic 7.4 in the interior, then it is clear that the ionization state of insulin will change as it passes through the membrane. Assuming anodal iontophoresis from a formulation at pH f4, then electromigration will drive the cationic insulin from the positive electrode and into the skin; however, as it crosses the barrier, it becomes progressively less cationic as the ambient pH rises, first becoming neutral at the pI, before becoming a molecular anion—at this point electromigration, theoretically, will reverse direction and the insulin will now move back towards the anode. In contrast, following cathodal iontophoresis from a solution at f7, the anionic insulin will become progressively more neutral as the pH falls to f5 in the outermost layers of the skin and may even become cationic, again being drawn back towards the cathodal compartment. In general, peptide candidates for iontophoretic delivery should have either a pI < 4 or a pI>8. Accordingly, the highest iontophoretic flux observed by Langkjaer et al. was for a sulfate-analog of monomeric porcine insulin which had a net _8 charge at pH 7.4 and a pI of f2.5[11].

6.2. Osteoporosis and Paget's disease

6.2.1. Calcitonin

Calcitonin is a 32 amino acid peptide with a molecular weight of f3500 Da; under physiological conditions it is positively charged. It is indicated for the treatment of Paget's disease and in the therapy of post-menopausal osteoporosis. Calcitonin is usually administered parenterally and, although nasal spray dosage forms are available, these result in low drug bioavailability. There has been considerable interest in the transdermal iontophoretic delivery of calcitonin and there are a number of reports in the literature describing in vitro and in vivo studies using various animal models. *Thysman et al.* investigated the pulsed iontophoretic delivery (2.5 kHz, 50% duty cycle) of human calcitonin using Pt-electrodes in a rat model and assessed its pharmacodynamic effect[11].

6.2.2. Human parathyroid hormone

Human parathyroid hormone (PTH), which contains 84 amino acids, has potential application in the treatment of osteoporosis since it promotes osteoblast growth. However, its pharmacological effect depends on the nature of the input profile. In healthy individuals, PTH is secreted by the parathyroid gland in a pulsatile manner and has an anabolic effect. However, it has been shown that continuous infusion of the peptide causes bone resorption. Based on these observations, *Suzuki et al.* conducted a detailed in vivo investigation into the pulsatile anodal iontophoretic delivery of hPTH(1-34), a pharmacologically active fragment of the intact peptide, in Sprague–Dawley rats, hairless rats and in beagles and compared the plasma concentration profiles and pharmacokinetic parameters to those observed after intravenous and subcutaneous injection. The anodal electrode compartment contained an aqueous conducting hydrogel, which was separated from the drug reservoir until use. The skin contact area was f9.6 cm2 and the iontophoretic current was applied for f60 min. Initial investigations into the effect of formulation parameters showed that, at a fairly modest constant current (0.1 mA cm^{-2}), the serum hPTH(1-34) levels showed a dose dependence and increased with increasing amounts of peptide in the patch; a 25-fold increase in drug loading (40–1000 Ag in the patch) produced a f15-fold increase in peak serum concentration. For a given drug load (200 Ag), doubling the current density from 0.05 to 0.1 mA cm^{-2}, caused an approximate

2-fold increase in peak serum levels. However, further increase in the current density to 0.15 mA cm^{-2}, produced a smaller increase, although the measured AUC was proportional to the current density. The mean transport rates upon application of a 200 mg dose at a current density of 0.1 mA cm^{-2} (applied for 60 min) were 6.7F0.3, 3.7F1.1 and 2.4F0.3 mg h^{-1} in Sprague–Dawley rats, beagles and hairless rats, respectively. A linear correlation was found between these absorption rates and the ratio of hair follicles, or skin porosity, to epidermal thickness. In subsequent experiments, Suzuki et al. demonstrated the feasibility of pulsatile iontophoretic administration and compared the anabolic effect hPTH(1-34), as evidenced by changes in bone mineral density, to that observed following subcutaneous injection. Their results suggested that a thrice-weekly threepulse protocol (3-30 min application of 0.1 mA cm^{-2} using a 120 Ag patch loading) was equivalent to daily subcutaneous injections of 5 Ag kg^{-1} in an ovariectomized rat model. Disodium etidronate is a member of the bisphosphonate family of drugs and is clearly not a peptide-based therapeutic but it is used in the treatment of Paget's disease. It is also indicated for the treatment of corticosteroid- induced osteoporosis. *Slough et al.* investigated the iontophoretic delivery of etidronate in vivo inpigs. A 5 cm^2 iontophoretic patch containing f10%etidronate and providing a current of 4 mA was able to deliver f2 mg of drug in 70 min. Comparison with an intravenous infusion of the drug (6 mg in 2 min), showed that, although the elimination kinetics were similar and that the area under the iontophoretic administration concentration–time profile approached f35% of that seen after IV infusion, the peak plasma concentration was f60-fold lower[12].

[7] COMPARING CLINICAL EFFICACY OF IONTOPHORETIC DELIVERY SYSTEMS

In these clinical studies, efficacy of treatment was usually the primary endpoint. However, an equally important parameter is the duration of current application required to obtain analgesia: a key objective in the optimization of an iontophoretic system is to maximize delivery while minimizing the current level.

This can be accomplished in a number of ways including optimization of the drug formulation and the use of different delivery profiles. The iontophoretic efficiency of a device can be described in terms of the total amount of charge that must be passed to obtain the desired clinical effect and quantified in units of milliamperes (mA) minutes—calculated by multiplying the electrical current and the application time. Clinical trials with the Vyteris system have shown efficacy at the 10 min time point with a current level of 1.77 mA (17.7 mA min). For the existing, first generation device, the same 10 min onset time requires a current level of 4.0 mA—equivalent to 40 mA min of charge transfer. Alternatively, at a 2.0 mA current level, the "fill on-site" device needs to be applied for 20 min[13].

[8] ADVANTAGES AND DISADVANTAGES

[8.1] Advantages

Iontophoresis provides for controlled delivery rates (through variations of current density, pulsed voltage, drug concentration and ionic strength). It eliminates gastrointestinal incompatibility, erratic absorption, and first pass metabolism. It reduces side effects and avoids the risks of infection, inflammation, and fibrosis associated with continuous injection or infusion since it is non-invasive. It enhances patient compliance with a convenient and non-invasive therapeutic regimen, and decreased dosing frequency. It improves efficacy by continuous release and decreases the total dose and dosing frequency.

The risk of infection is reduced because it's non-invasive. Drug solutions are delivered directly to the treatment sites without the disadvantages of injections or orally administered drugs. It provides pain-free for patients who are reluctant or unable to receive injections. It minimizes the potential for further tissue trauma that can occur with increased pressure from a fluid bolus injection. Drug dosage is accurately controlled by controlling the quantity of electrical current used to transfer the drug.

01. It is a non-invasive technique could serve as a substitute for chemical enhancers.

02. It eliminates problems like toxicity problem, adverse reaction formulation problems associated with presence of chemical enhancers in pharmaceuticals.

03. It may permit lower quantities of drug compared to use in TDDS, this may lead to fewer side effects.

04. TDDS of many ionized drug at therapeutic levels was precluded by their slow rate of diffusion under a concentration graduation, but iontophoresis enhanced flux of ionic drugs across skin under electrical potential gradient.

05. Iontophoresis prevent variation in the absorption of TDDS.

06. Eliminate the chance of over or under dosing by continuous delivery of drug programmed at the required therapeutic rate.

07. Provide simplified therapeutic regimen, leading to better compliance.

08. Permit a rapid termination of the modification, if needed, by simply by stopping drug input from the iontophoretic delivery system.

09. It is important in systemic delivery of peptide/protein based pharmaceuticals, which are very potent, extremely short acting and often require delivery in a circadian pattern to simulate physiological rhythm, eg. Thyrotropin releasing hormone, somatotropine, tissue plasminogen activates, inter ferons, enkaphaline, etc.

10. Provide predictable and extended duration of action.

11. Reduce frequency of dosage.

12. Self-administration is possible.

13. A constant current iontophoretic system automatically adjust the magnitude of the electric potential across skin which is directly proportional to rate of drug delivery and therefore, intra and inter-subject variability in drug delivery rate is substantially reduced. Thus, minimize inter and intra-patient variation.

14. An iontophoretic system also consists of a electronic control module which would allow for time varying of free-back controlled drug delivery.

15. Iontophoresis turned over control of local anesthesia delivery in reducing the pain of needle insertion for local anesthesia.

16. By minimizing the side effects, lowering the complexity of treatment and removing the need for a care to action, iontophoretic delivery improve adherence to therapy for the control of hypertension.

17. Iontophoretic delivery prevents contamination of drugs reservoir for extended period of time[14].

[8.2] Disadvantages

There is a possibility of burns if the electrodes are improperly used. The formation of undesirable vesicles and bullae in skin being treated can be avoided by periodically interrupting a unidirectional treatment current with a relatively short pulse of current in the opposite direction.

01. Iontophoretic delivery is limited clinically to those applications for which a brief drug delivery period is adequate.

02. An excessive current density usually results in pain.

03. Burns are caused by electrolyte changes within the tissues.

04. The safe current density varies with the size of electrodes.

05. The high current density and time of application would generate extreme pH, resulting in a chemical burn.

06. This change in pH may cause the sweat duct plugging perhaps precipitate protein in the ducts, themselves or cosmetically hyperhydrate the tissue surrounding the ducts.

07. Electric shocks may cause by high current density at the skin surface.

08. Possibility of cardiac arrest due to excessive current passing through heart.

09. Ionic form of drug in sufficient concentration is necessary for iontophoretic delivery.

10. High molecular weight 8000-12000 results in a very uncertain rate of delivery.

11. Patient should not have Iontophoresis if She is pregnant.

12. Patient should not have Iontophoresis if he/she have a cardiac pacemaker, have any metal orthopaedic implants.

13. Technique is not suitable for those patients who have fixed mouth braces[14].

[9] FACTORS AFFECTING IONTOPHORESIS

Variables affecting the iontophoresis include aspects of the current, the physicochemical properties of the drug, formulation factors, biological factors and electro-endo-osmotic flow.

[9.1] Current

Higher the intensity, greater the transport. The current can be direct, alternate or pulsed, and can have various waveforms, including square, sinusoidal, triangular and trapezoidal.

The more complex forms may not be of much advantage as direct current is most commonly used.

In a recent study, alternating current (AC) iontophoresis showed better results than conventional constant current DC iontophoresis. Constant conductance AC iontophoresis showed reduced flux drift and less skin to skin variability compared to conventional constant current DC iontophoresis.

Srinivasan et. al. suggested that increase in permeability of drug through skin may be more gradual than the increase in the current.

The relationship between the drug delivery rate (D) and current (I) follows the given question:

$$D = It \ M/Zf$$

Where, t is the fraction of current carried by drug ions or transference number, M is the molecular weight of drug ion, Z is the molecular charge per drug ion and F is Faraday's constant[15].

[9.2] Physicochemical variables

These include the charge, size, structure and lipophilicity of the drug. The drug should be water soluble, low-dose and ionizable with a high charge density. Smaller molecules are more mobile but large molecules are also iontophoresable.

1. **Characteristics of Penetrants:** The rate of penetration of substances through the intact skin depends on the size, charge, and configuration of molecules and relative solubility of the compound in lipid, water, in the Horney layer and on the vehicle in which the compound is presented to the skin. The iontophoresis gives uncertain drug delivery rate for an ionic solute of molecular weight 8000 to 12,000. For a negatively charged species, the size dependent flux enhancement neutralizes the influence of electric field. Conversely, positive charged species becomes increasingly important to effect the electric field as the size of permeant increases. *Pickal* reported that the flux enhancement ration for cations and neutral species in negative pores increases as the size of Penetrants increases.

2. **Polarisation:** Direct current can cause polarisation whilst pulsed current can decrease tissue polarization.

3. **Voltage:** The ionic flux due to an applied voltage drop across a membrane is based on the fundamental thermodynamic properties of the system. The diffusion of drug during iontophoresis follows Nerst-Plank equation. It states that the flux of the ionic drug due to applied electric filed is directly proportional to the voltage drop and charge of the ion. Masada et. al., demonstrated ionic flux of Tetraethyl ammonium bromide (TEAB) with varying voltage drop (0.125, 0.250, 0.250, 1.000). The enhancement factor for hairless mouse skin showed good agreement up to 0.5 volts and significantly higher at 1.0 volt due to skin damage but it is up to 0.25 V.

4. **Resistance:** The electrical resistance of the skin varies widely with iontophoretic drug delivery. The resistance of the skin during iontophoretic application was much lower on sweat pores, especially when they discharge sweat. A slight fall in resistance occurs when electrode was interested in to the epidermis.

5. **Electrodes:** The electrode materials used for iontophoretic delivery are to be harmless to the body and sufficiently flexible to apply closely to the body surface. The most common electrodes are aluminum foil, platinum and silver/silver chloride electrodes used for iontophoretic drug delivery. A better choice of electrode is silver/silver chloride because it minimizes electrolysis of water during drug delivery. The positioning of electrodes in reservoir depends on the charge of the

active drug. The distribution of drug within the skin depends on the size and position of electrodes. They are usually selected according to individuals needs. Larger electrode areas introduce the greater amounts of drug but lesser current density is tolerated to the skin in a non-linear manner. Metal electrodes touching to the skin produce burns with much lower current in composition to padded electrodes. A loose contact between the padded electrode and skin also produce burn due to uneven distribution of current. The safe current density varies with the size of electrodes.

6. **Temperature:** The penetration of drug through skin is affected by dual effect of both humidity and temperature. The iontophoretic delivery follows the Arhenious equation and enhances drug permeation with temperature.

7. **Frequency/Impedance:** The frequency of the applied current charges especially in man, variability of frequency dependent impedance of human skin ranges from 10 KHzs to 100 Khzs. The impedance of the skin decreases at higher frequencies less time is available to accumulate the charge on the skin surface during an applied pulse.The iontophoretic delivery of insulin decreases with increasing the frequency in the range of 50-2000 Hzs but Bagniefski and Burnett observed decrease in sodium ion flux with increase in frequency (10 Khzs). The theoretical relationship between impedance of skin and frequency follows this equation:

$$1/ZT = 1/ZR + 1/ZC.$$

8. **Wave Form:** The waveform also affects the iontophoretic delivery of drug. The insulin delivery was highest at sinusoidal waveform than square and triangular waveform.

9. **On/Off Ratio:** The on/off ratio of electricity effects the relative proportion of polarization and depolarization of skin, which results the efficiency of transdermal iontophoretic drug delivery. The number of on/off cycles in each second is shown as frequency. For example the on/off ration 1 : 1 at frequency 2000 Hzs (0.5 ms/cycle) provides 0.25 ms depolarization period and same time for the polarization.Liu et. al., suggested that the on /off ration of 1 : 1 at 2000 Hzs yields better glucose control for iontophoretic insulin delivery than 4:1, 8:1 on/off ration. Apparently, 1:4 and 8:1

rations, results a residue polarization the skin from the previous cycle which reduce the efficiency of insulin delivery.

10. **Duration of Application:** The transport of drug delivery depends on the duration of current applied in iontophoretic drug delivery. The iontophoretic penetration of drug linearly increased with increasing application time. The skin permeation of arginine vasopressin achieves higher plateau rate and in case of insulin delivery, 2-3 fold reduced the blood glucose levels with increase in duration of iontophoretic application[15].

[9.3] Biological factors

These factors involve the skin to which the electrodes are applied; its thickness, permeability, presence of pores, etc. Sweat glands are the most significant path for the conduction of charges into the skin. This was demonstrated by *Papa and Kligman*, when methylene blue introduced into the skin via iontophoresis entered sweat glands in a punctuate pattern and outlined the sweat pores.

01. **Species variation:** The vide differences in physical characteristics such as appendages per unit area, thickness and structural changes between human and laboratory rodent display a variation in penetration of drugs. The average penetration of drugs is in order of rabbit > rat > guineas pig > human. Human skin is very much less permeable than other rodents but iontophoretic delivery of drug is 7-fold greater in human skin consists of greater negative charge/or greater area fraction of negative pores. *Siddique et. al.*, observed that idiosyncrasy in hairless rats during the iontophoretic delivery of insulin[15].

[9.4] Formulation factors

These include the drug concentration, pH, ionic strength, and viscosity.

01. **Drug concentration:** Increasing drug concentrations results in greater drug delivery to a certain degree.

02. **Ionic strength:** If buffer ions are included, they compete with the drug for the delivery, decreasing the quantity of drug delivered, especially since buffer ions are generally smaller and more mobile than the larger active drug.

Higher ionic strength of the solution subjected to iontophoretic current resulted in decreased iontophoretic transport of the drug into the tissues as increase in ionic strength yields higher concentration of extraneous ions which compete for the electric current.

03. pH: The pH of the solution can be adjusted and maintained by larger molecules, such as ethanolamine: ethanolamine hydrochloride rather than the smaller hydrochloric acid and sodium hydroxide.

With metallic electrodes, shifts in pH are noted which can affect ionisation of the drug. pH changes in the tissue can use injury due to migration of hydronium and hydroxyl ions produced by electrolysis. Separate buffered electrolyte solutions can be used which can prevent flow of ions into the tissue.

Like charges repel each other while opposite charges attract. So to assist the positively charged lidocaine ions to be transported to the skin, the ionic form must be applied under a positively charged electrode which then moves to the cathode.

04. Viscosity: The migration of the drug is inversely related to the viscosity.

05. Ionised state of the drug: for eg. Lignocaine is mot effective iontophoretically at a pH range of 3.4-5.2. With iontophoresis transdermal permission is maximum at pH of 9.4 and above when it is mainly in the non-ionised state and at this pH, iontophoretic delivery is minimum.

06. Presence of extraneous ions: other ions of the some charge can decrease the iontophoretic delivery of the drug ions because these ions compete with the drug for the iontophoretic flux.

07. Buffer Systems: Buffer systems also affect the permeation of drugs by iontophoresis. It is important to optimize the concentration of buffer species in the system and should be sufficiently high to maintain good buffer capacity but should not reach an extent such that the current is mostly carried by the buffer species instead of drug special which may result the low efficiency of iontophoretic permeation[16.]

[10] ELECTRO-ENDO-OSMOSIS TRANSPORT

Drugs can also be transported via electro-endo-osmosis. When a current is applied, there is also a flow of water from the electrode reservoir into the skin. Any drug in solution, ionized or non-ionized, can follow the water flow into the skin. In this manner, some drugs that are not ionized can also be given iontophoretically. If only the non-ionized drug is to be given, it may be necessary to add a small quantity of sodium chloride to the solution for conductivity and to establish electro-endo-osmotic flow[17].

[11] EFFICIENCY OF DRUG DELIVERY

The efficiency of iontophoretic drug delivery can be defined as that fraction of all ions which cross the skin are drug ions which cross the skin for each mole of electrons flowing through the external circuit. This can be calculated from the slope of the plot of drug delivery rate ® versus current (I), which flows the given equation:

$$R = Ro + Fi. I$$

Where, Ro is the positive drug delivery using iontophoresis and Fi is the iontophoretic constant defined as the amount of drug (on a weight basis) delivered per uni-time per unit current[18].

[12] SYNERGISTIC MANNER OF DRUG DELIVERY

The penetration of drug through transdermal route can be achieved via the application of a combination of penetration enhancement technique. Several authors demonstrated the penetration of drugs (e.g. debutamine hydrochloride, azidothi-amidine) with the use of chemical enhancer (e.g. sod. Lauryl sulfate, decylmethyl sulfoxide) in combination of iontophoresis. The enhancement of drug through skin is greater with a combination technique, when the single technique is used. *Srinivasan et. al* explored the feasibility of synergism between the ethanol treated iontophoretic delivery of leuprolide and cholystokinin analogue. The penetration of tetracycline into tissue subject by the use of both Electro and phonophoresis were high than those obtained by the use of either Electro or phonophoresis. This invention relates to the use of certain transdermal flux enhancers in combination with iontophoresis for the topical administration of pharmaceutical agents[19].

Many pharmaceutical agents are ionized. As a result, in conventional topical drug delivery systems, they are unable to adequately penetrate the skin surface, and so do not reach the desired site of action at therapeutic concentrations. With such ionic drugs, this problem has been partially solved by the process of iontophoresis. By this means, it has been possible to enhance the localized delivery of drug to tissue (e.g., dermis, muscle, bone joints, and the like) which is at or near the site of application. By this means, it has also been possible to transport the drug into the blood stream, thus providing systemic delivery of drug to the entire body[19].

According to the process of iontophoresis, an electric potential is applied across a localized portion of body tissue as a drug containing solution is held against the skin in that localized area. Sufficient potential is applied so as to cause a small current to pass through the solution and the adjacent body tissue. In this manner, the drug is "phoresed" from the solution across the dermal barrier and into the local tissue (to produce high local tissue levels of the drug), or given enough time and other appropriate conditions, into the blood stream, whereby the drug is delivered systemically to more remote site(s) of action[19].

More recently, it has been shown in studies using mannitol that the flux of neutral, polar molecules is enhanced by iontophoresis, particularly in the presence of a cation such as Na$^+$. Thus the flux of a pharmaceutical agent which is not ionized or even capable of ionization can also be increased by the local application of an electric potential.

In the topical administration of pharmaceutical agents, iontophoresis is primarily limited by two interrelated factors: (1) Transport through the skin generally occurs via appendages (e.g., hair follicles, sweat glands, etc.) or small "pores", which represent only a fraction of the total skin surface area. Consequently, these pathways are exposed to a very high charge density relative to the total applied current, leading to irreversible changes or damage. (2) Since the rate of drug delivery is proportional to the applied current, the magnitude of delivery is severely limited by the problem described in (1) above[19].

As an alternative method for enhancing the transdermal flux of pharmaceutical agents, a variety of so-called penetration enhancers have been proposed for use as adjuncts in the topical administration of pharmaceutical agents.

Surprisingly, it has been found that the combination of iontophoresis with such transdermal flux enhancing agents leads to a synergistic effect in which flux across the dermal barrier is much higher than expected. This permits local and systemic delivery of a given amount of pharmaceutical agents by iontophoresis under much milder conditions of electrical potential and current density, avoiding the irreversible changes or damage to the skin.

This invention is directed to a method of treating a disease in a human or lower animal which comprises iontophoretic, topical administration of a pharmaceutical composition at reduced electric potential and current density. Accordingly, said composition comprises:

(a) a safe and effective amount of a pharmaceutical agent;

(b) an aqueous solvent; and

(c) a transdermal flux enhancing amount of a dermal penetration enhancer which is a 1-alkylazacycloheptan-2-one, said alkyl having from 8 to 16 carbon atoms, or a cis-olefin of the formula

$CH_3 (CH_2)x$ $CH.dbd.CH(CH_2)y$ R_3

where R_3 is $CH_2 OH$, $CH_2 NH_2$ or COR_4, and R_4 is OH or $(C_1 -C_4)$alkoxy, x and y are each an integer from 3 to 13 and the sum of x and y is from 10 to 16.

Preferred dermal penetration enhancers are cis-9-tetradecenoic acid, cis-6-pentadecenoic acid, cis-6-hexadecenoic acid, cis-9-hexadecenoic acid, cis-9-octadecenoic acid (oleic acid), cis-6-octadecenoic acid cis-11-octadecenoic acid, cis-12-octadecenoic acid, cis-5-eicosenoic acid, cis-9-eicosenoic acid, cis-11-eicosenoic acid, cis-14-eicosenoic acid, 1-decylazacycloheptan-2-one, 1-dodecylazacycloheptan-2-one or 1-tetradecylazacycloheptan-2-one. Most preferred is oleic acid.

The expression "aqueous solvent" refers to water itself as solvent, or a solvent which comprises, in addition to water, a water miscible organic solvent such as methanol, ethanol, isopropyl alcohol, propylene glycol, polyethylene glycol or glycerin.

This method is generally useful with neutral pharmaceutical agents which are not capable of ionization, particularly neutral agents which are polar in nature. However, this method finds its preferred use in the case of pharmaceutical agents which are ionized, or capable of ionization. This is true regardless of whether high drug levels are desired near the site of application (as is frequently the case, for example, in treating localized pain or inflammation, or a localized bacterial or fungal infection), or systemic delivery of the drug to more remote locations is desired (as is generally the case, for example, in the treatment of cardiovascular conditions, systemic infections, CNS conditions or diabetes).

This method is of particular value with

(a) analgesic or antiinflammatory agents used in the treatment of pain or an inflammatory disease, particularly aspirin, acetaminophen, indomethacin, ibuprofen, naproxen, the compound of the formula ##STR1## (generically named tenidap), piroxicam, and prodrugs of prioxicam of the formulas ##STR2## wherein R is $CH(R_1)OCOR_2$ or $CH(R_1)OCOOR_2$, R_1 is hydrogen or methyl and R_2 is $(C_1 -C_9)$ alkyl; and the pharmaceutically acceptable salts thereof;

(b) antifungal agents used in the treatment of a fungal infection, particularly fluconazole and tioconazole, and the pharmaceutically acceptable salts thereof;

(c) antibacterial agents used in the treatment of bacterial infections, particularly erythromycin, azithromycin, oxytetracycline, tetracycline, doxycycline, penicillin G, penicillin V, ampicillin and amoxicillin; and the pharmaceutically acceptable salts thereof; and

(d) agents used in the treatment of cardiovascular diseases, particularly nifedipine, amlodipine, prazosin, doxazosin and the compounds of the formula ##STR3## wherein X is O or C.dbd.O; and the pharmaceutically acceptable salts thereof.

The present method is also of particular value with the pharmaceutical agents sertraline (used in the treatment of depression) and insulin, glipizide, the compound of the formula ##STR4## and the compound of the formula ##STR5## (used in the treatment of diabetes); and the pharmaceutically acceptable salts thereof.

The present invention is readily carried out. Accordingly, a pharmaceutical agent, dissolved in an aqueous solvent in the presence of a conventional penetration enhancer, as defined above, is topically administered using a conventional iontophoretic device. In some instances, the solution of the pharmaceutical agent will also contain a pharmaceutically acceptable ionized salt, such as sodium chloride and/or buffering constituents. The presence of an ionic salt is particularly valuable when an ionizable pharmaceutical agent is administered at a pH at which the agent is largely in unionized form, and is generally essential when the pharmaceutical agent is not capable of ionization[19].

The dose of the drug, as well as the concentration of the drug in the aqueous solution and the volume of the solution, will, of course, depend upon the particular pharmaceutical agent administered and upon whether local or full systemic delivery of the drug is intended. In general, when systemic delivery is intended, the dose of the pharmaceutical agent will correspond approximately to that which is employed in the more conventional oral or parenteral route. Of course, when gastrointestinal absorption of a particular pharmaceutical agent is known to be poor, it will be possible to obtain high systemic levels of the pharmaceutical agent by the present iontophoretic methods with relatively lower doses of the pharmaceutical agent.

Typical unit dosages of pharmaceutical agents administered according to the present method, based upon use in an adult of about 50 to 80 Kg weight, are as follows: doxazosin, 1-25 mg; the compound of formula (I) above, 20-200 mg; aspirin, 200-1,000 mg; acetaminophen, 200-10,000 mg; indomethacin, 10-50 mg; ibuprofen, 200-1,000 mg; naproxen, 100-500 mg; the compound of the formula (III), 0.01-2 mg; piroxicam, 5-20 mg; fluconazole, 0.1-1 g; tioconazole, 0.1-1 g; erythromycin, 100-500 mg; azithromycin, 50-500 mg; oxytetracycline, 50-500 mg; tetracycline, 50-500 mg; doxycycline, 10-100 mg; penicillin G, 100,000-500,000 units; penicillin V, 100-500 mg; ampicillin, 100-500 mg; amoxicillin, 100-500 mg; nifedipine, 5-20 mg; amolodipine, 1-25 mg; prazosin, 0.25-1.25 mg; the compound of the formula (IV) wherein X is O, 1-10 mg; the compound of the formula (IV) wherein X is C.dbd.0, 1-10 mg; insulin, 50-1,000 units; glipizide, 2.5-10 mg; the compound of the formula (V), 1-20 mg; the compound of the formula (VI), 1-20 mg; and sertraline, 1-20 mg. However, in particular circumstances, doses outside of these ranges will be used at the discretion of the attending physician.

When high localized concentrations of the desired drug are desired, the pharmaceutical agent will be administered iontophoretically, generally for a relatively short period of time, with the electric potential applied across the site where a high local concentration of the agent is desired; for example, with analgesics at the site of pain, with antiinflammatory agents at the site of inflammation, and with antibacterials or antifungals at the site of a localized infection.

On the other hand, when full systemic delivery of the pharmaceutical agent is desired, the site of administration is less critical. However, the site should be well supplied with blood vessels, so that the agent readily reaches the blood stream, which rapidly removes it from the site of administration and distributes it throughout the body. Generally, systemic delivery will require longer periods of iontophoresis, permitting maximal absorption and systemic delivery of the pharmaceutical agent[19].

According to this method, the concentration of penetration enhancer employed is generally in the range of 0.01-5% (w/v), i.e., similar to the levels used absent iontophoresis. Preferred levels are generally in the range of about 0.1 to 1%. However, iontophoretic administration of pharmaceutical agents, according to the present method, is generally achieved under much milder conditions of electric potential and current density, avoiding irreversible changes or damage to the skin which can occur at higher potentials and/or current densities.

The synergistic effect of iontophoresis and a skin penetration agent in moving a pharmaceutical agent across the dermal barrier is demonstrated by iontophoresis experiments detailed below.

This invention is illustrated by the following examples. However, it should be understood that the invention is not limited to the specific details of these examples.

EXAMPLE 1

Influence of Oleic Acid on the Transport of Sodium Ion Across the Dermal Barrier by Iontophoresis.

Diffusion cells were used in all transport studies. A 0.64-cm^2 area of tissue membrane was exposed to the donor and receptor compartments of each diffusion cell. The reservoirs were magnetically stirred, water jacketed, and had volumes of 3.0 mL. Temperature control (37°±0.2° C.) was provided by a constant temperature bath (Haake A80) with an external circulator (American Scientific Products, McGaw Park, Ill.). Electodes were made by lightly sanding Ag wires (99.9% purity; 4 cm×1.0 mm) and placing them in a 1M HCl solution for 10 minutes at 50° C. The Ag wires were then rinsed with distilled water and plated with AgCl by applying a current of 0.20 mA (both the cathode and anode were Ag wires) through a 0.5M KCl solution for 12 hours. Subsequently, the Ag--AgCl wires were plated with platinum black by passing a 100-mA current (the cathode was the Ag--AgCl electrode and the anode was a Pt wire of 99.99% purity) for 3-5 minutes through a solution containing 0.66 mM Pb(C2 H3 O2)2 and 0.073M H2 PtCl6. The electrodes were positioned approximately 2 cm from either side of the tissue membrane, with the anode placed on the epidermal side and the cathode on the dermal side. The constant current required in the iontophoretic experiments was obtained from a programmable constant current source (model 224; Keithley Instruments, Inc., Cleveland, Ohio). Slight pH changes during iontophoresis were monitored (Digi-pH-ase LED pH meter equipped with an extra-slender neck, glass-body combination electrode, Cole Parmer, Ill.) and corrected for by the addition of microliter amounts of 1M HCl or 1M NaOH solutions. These additions changed the overall Na^+ and Cl^- concentrations by a few percent at most. By this technique the pH was kept to within ±0.1 pH unit of 7.4.

Excised porcine skin from freshly slaughtered pigs was obtained using a Padgett electrodermatome set at 0.8 mm thickness. A thickness of 0.8 mm was chosen because it could be reproducibly obtained with the dermatome and because it resulted in specimens which were generally intact. Each piece of tissue was examined for any gross morphological damage such as tears or holes under a stereomicroscope, at a magnification of ×30 and ×60 using both transmitted and reflected light for illumination. All tissue was obtained within 24 hours after death, positioned dermal side down on a piece of filter paper soaked with 0.9% NaCl, placed in a petri-dish, stored at 4° C., and used approximately 12 hours later.

All chemicals were used as received and all solutions were made using distilled water which had been passed through a Barnstead PCS water purification system (which contains charcoal filter and a mixed-bed ion exchange resin, the resulting water having a pH of 6-8 and a resistance of 14-18 Mohm/cm). Transport studies were carried out using buffer solutions which were 3:2 by volume mixtures of 0.13M NaCl in 25 mM HEPES buffer and ethanol. All buffers were degassed prior to use by sonicating the buffer at 40° C. under reduced pressure in order to prevent bubble formation on the tissue, which could result in artifactual transport results. Radiotracer solutions were made up in the buffer 22 Na^+ (0.3 μCi/mL) obtained from NEN Research Products (Boston, Mass.). In those experiments employing oleic acid, this compound was present at a level of 0.25% w/v in the buffer solution.

Transport studies were performed by mounting the excised tissue in the diffusion cell, placing plain buffer solution in the chamber adjacent to one side of the tissue, adding buffer containing tracer to the other chamber, inserting electrodes (if required), and turning on the magnetic stirrers. The starting time was defined as the time when the current was turned on, with samples being taken at 0.75-1.5 hour intervals for 8.25 hours. Samples of 2 mL were obtained by disconnecting the current source, removing the entire contents of the receiving cell, rinsing the receiving cell with fresh buffer, replacing with 3 mL of fresh buffer, and reconnecting the electrodes and current source. The 22 Na^+ samples were counted in a auto-gamma scintillation spectrometer 5236 (Packard Instrument Company, Downers Grove, Ill.). The mean total counts obtained had standard errors of the mean (SEM) which were less than $\pm 5\%$ of the mean (n=3) except for the passive diffusion samples which were greater than $\pm 5\%$.

Fluxes were calculated from the quantity of radioisotope transferred per unit time and the specific radioactivity in the donor compartment. (Control experiments showed that the free solution specific activity of the isotope in the donor chamber remained approximately constant throughout the course of an experiment. This implies that loss of isotope through transport into the receiving chamber or through absorption of isotope onto the glass or the electrodes was negligible.) The fluxes were expressed per unit area by dividing the flux by the surface area of the tissue (0.64 cm^2). These fluxes were defined to occur at a time equal to the total elapsed time minus one-half the collection time interval.

For the experiments whose results are shown in Table I, the anode and the Na^+ tracer were placed in the chamber facing the dermal side of the tissue. Control experiments show no significant passive flux of Na^+ absent electric current or oleic acid.

The synergistic effect of iontophoresis coupled with oleic acid is demonstrated by the data in Table II. The expected flux, which is the sum of the flux resulting from current alone and oleic acid alone, is generally well below that observed with combined use of current and oleic acid.

TABLE I

Average Na+ Flux (μmol/cm2 /h)

Time (h)	OAa alone	Current alone 0.25 μAmp	Current alone 100 μAmp	OAa + Current 0.25 μAmp	OAa + Current 100 μAmp
0.75	0.1	0.5	2.0	0.8	3.1
2.25	0.3	0.9	3.8	1.6	6.0
3.75	0.8	1.0	4.5	1.7	6.5
5.25	1.0	1.0	5.0	2.1	7.4
6.75	1.3	1.3	5.0	2.5	7.5
8.25	1.7	1.2	5.2	2.6	8.2

a Oleic Acid, 0.25%

TABLE II

Additive Na+ Versus Observed Flux

with Oleic Acid and Current

Time   25 μAmp   100 μAmp

(h)   Calcd. Observed Calcd.

Observed

Time (h)	25 μAmp Calcd.	25 μAmp Observed	100 μAmp Calcd.	100 μAmp Observed
0.75	0.6	0.8	2.1	3.1
2.25	1.2	1.6	4.1	6.0
3.75	1.8	1.7	5.3	6.5
5.25	2.0	2.1	6.0	7.4
6.75	2.6	2.5	6.3	7.5
8.25	2.9	2.6	6.9	8.2

EXAMPLE 2

Treatment of Hypertension with Doxazosin Using Iontophoresis and Oleic Acid

A. Apparatus--An electrical device capable of generating a constant current of from 0.1 to 9.0 mA using a power source of up to 10 volts. Two electrodes, anode and cathode made of appropriate material (e.g., Ag/AgCl or platinum). The anode or positive electrode is a pliable reservoir (3-5 ml) with a semipermeable porous membrane for placement next to the skin. The cathode or return electrode is filled with a conductive gel.

B. Drug Solutions--Doxazosin (2-20 mg, as the mesylate salt) is dissolved in a 3-5 ml volume of 20-70% (v/v) ethanol vehicle. The vehicle also contains 5-100 mM of a phosphate buffer at pH 3-5 and 0.1-1% (w/v) of oleic acid.

C. Administration--The above solution of doxazosin is filled into the anode reservoir. The anode is a fixed to the surface of the chest with adhesive while the return electrode is placed on an adjacent area. 0.1-5 mA of current is applied for 10-90 minutes until systemic delivery of the drug is sufficient to reduce blood pressure to the desired level.

EXAMPLE 3

Treatment of Muscle or Arthritic Joint Pain and Inflammation with Piroxicam Using Iontophoresis and Oleic Acid.

A. Background--This type of therapy is applicable to acute flare-ups or injury and is used in place of or in conjunction with oral therapy to enhance drug levels locally at the intended site.

B. Apparatus--Same as the preceding example, except that the cathode (-) is the drug electrode and the anode (+) is the return electrode.

C. Drug Solutions--Same as the preceding example, except that 1 mg/ml of piroxicam concentration at pH 7.4 is used.

D. Administration--Same as the preceding example, except electrodes are placed adjacent to site of injury or pain/inflammation[19].

[13] REVERSE IONTOPHORESIS

The application of an electric current across the skin is used to extract a substance of interest from within or beneath the skin to the surface for testing. In vivo and in vitro methods have shown that the approach can be used to monitor the subdermal concentration variation of glucose and provide a non-invasive technique by which a diabetic can monitor the fluctuation of blood sugar[20].

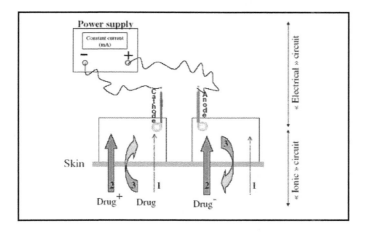

[14] IONTOPHORETIC DEVICES

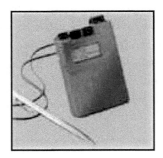

The main manufacturing concerns as in any equipment should include safety, convenience, reliability and reproducibility of the device. The components of the equipments are:

- An microprocessor controlled.
- A low voltage direct current generator,the power source it runs on a single 9-volt alkaline battery.

- Lead wires consisting of a positive lead and a negative lead. One unit has dual channel capacity, enabling treatment of 2 different sites at once. (2 channel device- allow to treat 2 different sites or use drug solutions of different polarities at the same time)
- Electrodes, consisting a buffered drug containment electrode for delivery of the drug[21].

[15] APPLICATIONS OF IONTOPHORESIS

Iontophoresis has been used for the treatment of various dermatologic conditions. The majority of published studies are either uncontrolled series or anecdotal observations. Earlier, simple ions and heavy metals were the most frequently used drugs, but over the last 30 years interest has shifted toward the use of iontophoresis as a drug delivery system for a wide variety of medications, ranging from steroids to antibiotics to local anesthetics[21].

[15.1] Ulcers

Iontophoresis has been used for the treatment of patients with ischemic leg ulcers. The effect of histamine iontophoresis on ulcers was studied by *Abramson et al*. Complete healing was reported in four of the five patients. Cornwell reported a patient with ischemic ulcer who responded to iontophoresis with solution of zinc oxide.

[15.2] Fungal infection

There are reports of the successful treatment of dermatophytosis with the use of copper sulfate iontophoresis and of sporotrichosis with potassium iodide iontophoresis. Copper-iontophoresis for fungal infection and male contraception, zinc for ulcers, iodine for reduction of scar tissues, iron/titanium oxide for tattoo removal.

[15.3] Viral Infections

(1) **Warts:** There is a report of the successful treatment of plantar warts with sodium salicylate iontophoresis.

(2) **Herpes simplex:** *Gangarosa* reported that iontophoretic application of idoxuridine was effective in aborting episodes of herpes simplex. *Lekas* reported relief of discomfort and reduction of healing time of herpes simplex lesions in a controlled trial using iontophoresis with idoxuridine.

[15.4] Cystic fibrosis

In the diagnosis of cystic fibrosis to increase sweating by pilocarpine and confirm diagnosis by the concentration of sodium and chloride in the sweat.

[15.5] Aphthous stomatitis

In a small group of patients with aphthous stomatitis, iontophoresis of triamcinolone acetonide showed immediate relief of discomfort in the prodromal stage, but for lesions beyond the prodromal stage relief was not achieved until after 36 hours.

[15.6] Lichen planus

In an uncontrolled series, *Gangarosa* reported iontophoresis with methyl prednisolone for erosive lichen planus, which healed with fibrosis.

[15.7] Hyperhidrosis

The most successful application of iontophoresis is for the treatment of hyperhidrosis. The basis for such treatment and its practical aspects have been well described. Currently, the most commonly used conducting medium is tap water because it is safe and effective. Anticholinergic compounds (e.g. poldine methyl sulfate, glycopyrronium bromide, and atropine) have a longer lasting effect than water, but the side effects of systemic anticholinergic blockade have prevented their wide acceptance.

The efficacy and safety of tap water iontophoresis is well documented, but its mechanism of action remains unknown. The most widely accepted hypothesis is that sweating is inhibited by mechanical blockage of the sweat ducts at the stratum corneum level, the depth and severity of the damage being dose-related. Stripping off the stratum corneum relieves the blockage and restores sweating. More recent work by *Hill et al* casts doubt on this theory. They examined, by light and electron microscopy, sweat glands from the palm of a patient with hyperhidrosis before and after treatment and found no changes. No side effects when compared to anti- cholinergics[22, 23].

[15.8] Anesthesia

Otolaryngologists have used iontophoresis of local anesthetics for anesthesia of the middle ear, and dentists, for anesthesia of the oral mucosa. Anesthesia of the skin can be achieved with the use of a variety of positive and negative controls, including iontophoresis of epinephrine and lidocaine separately, and topical administration of lidocaine and epinephrine. Skin anesthesia is best obtained with solutions containing 1% and 4% lidocaine and between 1/10,000 and 1/50,000 epinephrine. Iontophoresis of anesthetics may be useful especially for pediatric patients.

[15.9] Ophthalmology

Iontophoretic induction of various drugs like atropine, scopolamine, sulfadiazine, fluorescein, gentamycin etc.

[15.10] ENT

For providing anaesthesia of the external ear canal and middle ear and in maxillo facial prosthetics surgeries.

[15.11] Dentistry

To prevent dentin hypersensitivity and for providing local anaesthetic for multiple tooth extraction.

[15.12] Neurophysiological and Neuropharmacological studies

As a research tool, micro-iontophoresis can be used to study neuro muscular junction, peripheral and central nervous system and smooth muscle preparations.

[15.13] Delivery of drugs

Antihypertensives, anti-diabetics, anti-rheumatoids, hormones, vasodilators: Metaprolol, propranolol, insulin, methylcholine, bleomycin, steroids have all been introduced iontophoretically.

[15.14] Musculo skeletal disorders

Magnesium sulphate for bursitis, Calcium for myopathy, Silver for c/c osteomyelitis, local anaesthetics and steroids into elbow, shoulder and knee joints[23].

[15.15] Cardiology

Iontophoretic transmyocardial drug delivery of anti-arrhythmic drugs which would avoid high systemic toxic levels is being done in animals[23].

[15.16] For relief of pain

- Iontophoretic histamine delivery as counter-irritant.
- In painless venipuncture.
- For post-operative pain relief.
- For iontophoretic delivery of local anaesthetics for referred pain.
- Anti-inflammatory drug delivery[24].

[15.17] Miscellaneous uses

Hyperkeratosis with fissuring of palms and soles: Iontophoresis with 5-10% aqueous solution of sodium salicylate showed improvement within a period of 3-4 weeks (6-8 sittings of 10-15 minutes each).

(1) Vitiligo: In an uncontrolled study, iontophoresis with meladine solution 1% in patients with vitiligo showed marked repigmentation.

(2) Scleroderma: In one trial, iontophoresis with hyaluronidase led to increased skin softness and flexibility of tissues and decreased cold sensitivity. On termination of therapy, cold sensitivity returned in a week but the improvement in skin softness and flexibility persisted for three months. In scleroderma, for iontophoretic delivery of hyaluronidase.

(3) Lymphedema: Iontophoresis with hyaluronidase has also been successfully used in the treatment of lymphedema of the limbs.

(4) Patch testing: *Wahlberg* reported encouraging results with the use of iontophoresis as a complement to ordinary patch testing in the investigation of obscure cases of contact eczema. With iontophoresis, the test substances are administered rapidly and they migrate through the epidermis down into the dermis. Additionally, the disadvantages of the traditional patch test procedure, such as prolonged wearing of the test strips, are eliminated.

(5) Sweat test: Iontophoresis was also used for the diagnosis of cystic fibrosis by the sweat test. Iontophoresis with pilocarpine causes rapid sweating for minutes.

Other applications of iontophoresis include introduction of "artificial skin pigment" (iron oxide and titanium oxide) into the skin, iodine iontophoresis to reduce scar tissue, histamine in allergy testing and administration of antibiotics (penicillin) in burn patients.

This is an area which has wide scope for expansion. We have seen the varied applications and the potential for improvement for this method of drug delivery. Further research is required to perfect this technique. There are several devices now available in all sizes and shapes to suit individual needs and ensure absolute safety. With even pencil shaped transdermal applicators now available for self administration, iontophoresis may prove to be an important alternative method of drug delivery in the near future[25, 26].

[16] PRECAUTIONS

- keep patients hands or feet in the baths once treatment has started this will receive an unpleasant electric shock, which is not dangerous.

- Avoid contact with the metal plate electrodes to avoid any burns by not pressing down on the plastic grills too hard.

- Remove all jewellery and nail polish including rings, bracelets, watches and body piecing. If any rings cannot be removed, they must be covered with tape to avoid burns.

- Cover any cuts or open lesions to hands or feet that are to be treated with petroleum jelly (white soft paraffin) to prevent tenderness or pain.

- Patient must inform the staff if he has cardiac pacemakers, metal orthopaedic implants, and if female she should tell that whether pregnant or not.

- Please inform staff if patient has any cuts or lesions to his hands and / or feet[27].

[17] POSSIBLE SIDE EFFECTS

- Patient may experience pins and needles sensation; however, it is not painful. The treatment can cause a tingling sensation to hands/feet (or even limbs).

- Very rarely, mild burns and spasms of electrical current can occur. These are not painful or dangerous.

- Iontophoresis is not a permanent solution to the problem and further treatments may be needed at a later stage. Equipment can be purchased for maintenance treatment at home. The address of a supplier is included at the end of this leaflet.

- If patient suffer from eczema this treatment may cause this to flare.

- If patient have eczema, it may worsen the condition. He could suffer some slight bruising if the intensity of the treatment is too great.

- Moderate temporary thickening of the skin (hyperkeratosis) could occur if the treatment sessions are too frequent[28, 29].

[18] DURATION OF TREATMENT

The treatment consists of seven (20 or 30 minute) sessions over a four-week period. Appointments must be kept to the days stated below, so its the duty of the patient to please inform staff if he is likely to be away for any of this period, as it will affect your treatment. In this case, it would be best to start treatment at a later date.

- Week 1 - Day 1, 2 & 4 (Tuesday, Wednesday & Friday)

- Week 2 - Day 7 & 10 (Monday & Thursday)

- Week 3 - Day 15 (Tuesday)

- Week 4 - Day 22 (Tuesday)[30]

[19] CONCLUSION AND FUTURE PERSPECTIVES

Transdermal drug delivery by means of ion-tophoresis can be an excellent tool to deliver suitable drugs 'on-demand' especially for suitable multi-factorial diseases such as Parkinson's disease. With apomorphine it could 'be shown' in a first study Parkinson patients that with a tolerable patch size between 50 and 80 cm , therapeutic plasma levels can be achieved albeit at the lower level of therapeutic effect. The use of suitable chemical enhancers or vesicular formulations may be an interesting tool in combination with the electrically enhanced transdermal delivery of apomorphine to both increase the therapeutic efficacy of apomorphine and to reduce the patch size. A second study with Parkinson patients with iontophoretic delivery of apomorphine is currently being performed using optimized surfactant formulations for pretreatment before iontophoresis occurs.

The most interesting feature of using iontophoresis for controlled drug delivery is that the Parkinson patient can directly control the needed amount of apomorphine by increasing or decreasing the drug input in order to achieve optimal drug therapy with a minimum of toxic side effects. Furthermore, the typical features of Parkinson's disease such bradykinesia, akinesia and tremor could be used to directly monitor the needed drug input by means of chip sensors which are able to directly measure the most important Parkinson disease parameters and to regulate the drug input. Such a system would be the very first closed loop system monitoring not pharmacokinetic data but more importantly pharmacodynamic effect of Parkinson's disease. This scenario is more feasible as skin irritation and toxicity studies have proven that iontophoresis is the safe route of treatment.

In general terms, the future perspective of iontophoresis are miniaturization of the devices reducing the costs of the treatment by producing diposable drug containing patches developing high energy batteries for microcomputers to be used as hardware. Also the design of a suitable charged drug of high potency will increase the use and versatility of iontophoresis devices including targeting of antigens to Langerhans cells in the skin.

[20] REFERENCES

1. A. Naik, Y.N. Kalia, R.H. Guy, Transdermal drug delivery: overcoming the skin's barrier function, Pharm. Sci. Technol. Today 3 (2000) 318– 326.

2. R.O. Potts, M.L. Francoeur, The influence of stratum corneum morphology on water permeability, J. Invest. Dermatol. 96 (1991) 495–499.

3. Y.N. Kalia, V. Merino, R.H. Guy, Transdermal drug delivery. Clinical aspects, Dermatol. Clin. 16 (1998) 289–299.

4. C. Cullander, G. Rao, R.H. Guy, Why silver/silver chloride? Criteria for iontophoresis electrodes, Prediction Percutaneous Penetration 3B (1993) 381-390.

5. J.B. Phipps, R.V. Padmanabhan, G.A. Lattin, Iontophoretic delivery of model inorganic and drug ions, J. Pharm. Sci. 78 (1989) 365–369.

6. B.H. Sage, J.E. Riviere, Model systems in iontophoresis transport efficacy, Adv. Drug Deliv. Rev. 9 (1992) 265–287.

7. R.R. Burnette, Iontophoresis, in: J. Hadgraft, R.H. Guy (Eds.), Transdermal Drug Delivery: Developmental Issues and Research Initiatives, vol. 35, Marcel Dekker, New York, 1989, pp. 247– 291.

8. G.B. Kasting, Theoretical models for iontophoretic delivery, Adv. Drug Deliv. Rev. 9 (1992) 177– 199.

9. http://www.empi.com/b/b4_1.html.

10. http://www.dcu.ie/~best/idd.htm.

11. http://www.webn.com/WEVR/V2N1/Innovations/Inovations 2.html

12. http://www.unipr.it/arpa/dipfarm/erasmus/erasm14.html.

13. P.G. Green, M. Flanagan, B. Shroot, R. Guy, Iontophoretic drug delivery, in: K. Waiters and J. Hadgkraft (Eds.), Dermal Drug Delivery, Marcel Dekker, New York, 1993, pp. 297-319.

14. M. R. Prausnitz, V. G. Bose, R. Langer, J. C. Weaver, Electroporation of mammalian skin: a mechanism to enhance transdermal drug delivery. Proc. Natl. Acad. Sci. USA 90 (1993) 10504-10508.

15. P.W. Wertz, D.T. Downing, Stratum corneum: biological and biochemical considerations, In: J. Hadgraft and R. H. Guy (Eds.) Transdermal Drug Delivery. Developmental Issues and Research Initiatives, Marcel Dekker, New York, 1989, pp. 1-22.

16. R. O. Potts, M. L. Freancoeur, Lipid biophysics of water loss through the skin, Proc. Natl. Acad. Sci. USA 87 (1990) 3871-3873.

17. K.A. Waiters, Penetration enhancers and their use in transdermal therapeutic systems, in: J. Hadgraft and R.H. Guy (Eds.), Transdermal Drug Delivery: Developmental Issues and Research Initiatives. Marcel Dekker, New York (1989), 197- 246.

18. M. Kazim, C. Webber, L. G. Strausberg LaForet, J. Nicholson and K. Reemtstma, Treatment of diabetes in mice with topical application of insulin to the skin Diabetes 33 (1984) 181A.

19. W.J. Albery and J. Hadgraft, Percutaneous absorption: in vivo experiments, J. Pharm. Pharmacol. 31 (1979) 140-147.

20. R.B. Stoughton, Enhanced percutaneous penetration with 1 dodecyllazacycloheptan-2-one, Arch. Dermatol. 118 (1982) 474---477.

21. E.R. Cooper, Alterations in skin permeability, in: Y.W. Chien (Ed.), Transdermal Controlled Systemic Medication, M. Dekker, New York, 1987, pp. 83-92.

22. H.E. Bodde, J. Verhoeven and L.M.J. van Driel, The skin compliance of transdermal drug delivery systems, Crit. Rev. Ther. Drug. Cart. Syst. 6 (1989) 87-96.

23. M. Mezei, Liposomes as a skin delivery system, in: D.D. Breimer and P. Speiser (Eds.), Topics in Pharmacological Science, Elsevier, Amsterdam, 1985, pp. 345-358.

24. G. Cevc, G. Blume, Lipid vesicles penetrate into intact skin owing to the transdermal osmotic gradients and hydration force. Biochim. Biophys. Acta 1104 (1992) 226-232.

25. H. Schreier, J. Bouwstra, Liposomes and niosomes as topical drug carriers: dermal and transdermal drug delivery J. Control.Release 30 (1994) 1-15.

26. G. Cevc, Lipid properties as a basis for the modelling and design of liposome membranes, in: G. Gregoriadis (Ed.), Liposome Technology, 2nd ed., CRC Press, Boca Raton, FL, 1992, pp. 1-36.

27. G. Cevc, editor. Phospholipids Handbook. Marcel Dekker, New York, Basel, Hong Kong (1993).

28. B.R. Meyer, H.L. Katzeff, J. Eschbach, J. Trimmer, S.R. Zacharias, S. Rosen, and D. Sibalis, Transdermal delivery of human insulin to albino rabbits using electrical current, Amer. J. Med. Sci. 297 (1989) 321-325.

29. O. Siddiqui, Y. W. Chien, Nonparenteral administration of peptide and protein drugs, Critical Reviews in Therapeutic Drug Cartier Systems 3 (1987) 195-208.

30. M. Mishima, S. Okada, Y. Wakita, and M. Nakano, Promotion of nasal absorption of insulin by glycyrrhetinic acid derivatives. J. Pharmacobio.-Dynam. 12 (1989) 31-36.

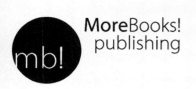
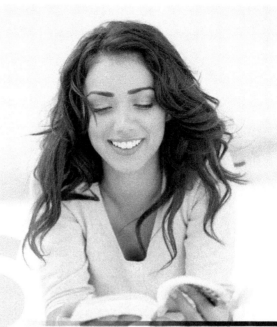

Lightning Source UK Ltd.
Milton Keynes UK
UKHW041943021218
333358UK00001B/83/P

9 783848 489084